COMBINING FORM

aden/o

EXAMPLE: aden/oma

COMBINING FORM

cancer/o, carcin/o

EXAMPLE: cancer/ous

COMBINING FORM

chlor/o

EXAMPLE: chlor/oma

COMBINING FORM

chrom/o

EXAMPLE: xanth/o/chrom/ic

COMBINING FORM

cyan/o

EXAMPLE: cyan/osis

COMBINING FORM

cyt/o

EXAMPLE: cyt/o/logy

COMBINING FORM

epitheli/o

EXAMPLE: epitheli/oma

COMBINING FORM

erythr/o

EXAMPLE: erythr/o/cyte

cancer

gland

color

green

cell

blue

red

epithelium

eti/o

EXAMPLE: eti/o/logy

fibr/o

EXAMPLE: fibr/o/sarcoma

gno/o

EXAMPLE: pro/gno/sis

hist/o

EXAMPLE: hist/o/logy

iatr/o

EXAMPLE: iatr/o/genic

kary/o

EXAMPLE: kary/o/plasm

lei/o

EXAMPLE: lei/o/my/oma

leuk/o

EXAMPLE: leuk/o/cyte

fiber

cause (of disease)

tissue

knowledge

nucleus

physician, medicine
(also means treatment)

white

smooth

lip/o

EXAMPLE: lip/oma

melan/o

EXAMPLE: melan/oma

my/o

EXAMPLE: my/o/pathy

neur/o

EXAMPLE: neur/oma

onc/o

EXAMPLE: onc/o/logist

organ/o

EXAMPLE: organ/ic

path/o

EXAMPLE: path/o/genic

rhabd/o

EXAMPLE: rhabd/o/my/oma

black

fat

nerve

muscle

organ

tumor, mass

rod-shaped, striated

disease

sarc/o

EXAMPLE: sarc/oma

somat/o

EXAMPLE: somat/o/plasm

system/o

EXAMPLE: system/ic

viscer/o

EXAMPLE: viscer/al

xanth/o

EXAMPLE: xanth/o/chrom/ic

dia-

EXAMPLE: dia/gno/sis

dys-

EXAMPLE: dys/plasia

hyper-

EXAMPLE: hyper/plasia

body

flesh, connective tissue

internal organs

system

through, complete

yellow

above, excessive

painful, abnormal, difficult, labored

PREFIX

hypo-

EXAMPLE: hypo/plasia

PREFIX

meta-

EXAMPLE: meta/stasis

PREFIX

neo-

EXAMPLE: neo/plasm

PREFIX

pro-

EXAMPLE: pro/gno/sis

SUFFIX

-al, -ic, -ous

EXAMPLE: epitheli/al

SUFFIX

-cyte

EXAMPLE: erythr/o/cyte

SUFFIX

-gen

EXAMPLE: carcin/o/gen

SUFFIX

-genic

EXAMPLE: carcin/o/genic

after, beyond, change

below, incomplete, deficient, under

before

new

cell

pertaining to

producing, originating, causing

substance or agent that produces or causes

-logist

EXAMPLE: onc/o/logist

-logy

EXAMPLE: onc/o/logy

-megaly

EXAMPLE: organ/o/megaly

-oid

EXAMPLE: cyt/oid

-oma

EXAMPLE: fibr/oma

-osis

EXAMPLE: cyan/osis

-pathy

EXAMPLE: somat/o/pathy

-plasia

EXAMPLE: hyper/plasia

study of

one who studies and treats (specialist, physician)

resembling

enlargement

abnormal condition (means **increase** when used with blood cell word roots)

tumor, swelling

condition of formation, development, growth

disease

SUFFIX

-plasm

EXAMPLE: neo/plasm

SUFFIX

-sarcoma

EXAMPLE: aden/o/sarcoma

SUFFIX

-sis

EXAMPLE: pro/gno/sis

SUFFIX

-stasis

EXAMPLE: meta/stasis

COMBINING FORM

anter/o

EXAMPLE: anter/o/poster/ior

COMBINING FORM

caud/o

EXAMPLE: caud/al

COMBINING FORM

cephal/o

EXAMPLE: cephal/ic

COMBINING FORM

dist/o

EXAMPLE: dist/al

malignant tumor

growth, substance, formation

control, stop, standing

state of

tail (downward)

front

away (from the point of attachment of a body part)

head (upward)

COMBINING FORM

dors/o

EXAMPLE: dors/al

COMBINING FORM

infer/o

EXAMPLE: infer/ior

COMBINING FORM

later/o

EXAMPLE: later/al

COMBINING FORM

medi/o

EXAMPLE: medi/al

COMBINING FORM

poster/o

EXAMPLE: poster/ior

COMBINING FORM

proxim/o

EXAMPLE: proxim/al

COMBINING FORM

super/o

EXAMPLE: super/ior

COMBINING FORM

ventr/o

EXAMPLE: ventr/al

below

back

middle

side

near (the point
of attachment of a
body part)

back, behind

belly (front)

above

bi-

EXAMPLE: bi/later/al

uni-

EXAMPLE: uni/later/al

-ad

EXAMPLE: cephal/ad

-ior

EXAMPLE: poster/o/anter/ior

aut/o

EXAMPLE: dermat/o/aut/o/plasty

bi/o

EXAMPLE: bi/opsy

coni/o

EXAMPLE: dermat/o/coni/osis

crypt/o

EXAMPLE: onych/o/crypt/osis

one

two

pertaining to

toward

life

self

hidden

dust

cutane/o, derm/o, dermat/o

EXAMPLE: dermat/o/logy

heter/o

EXAMPLE: dermat/o/heter/o/plasty

hidr/o

EXAMPLE: hidr/aden/itis

kerat/o

EXAMPLE: kerat/o/genic

myc/o

EXAMPLE: onych/o/myc/osis

necr/o

EXAMPLE: necr/osis

onych/o, ungu/o

EXAMPLE: sub/ungu/al

pachy/o

EXAMPLE: pachy/derm/a

other

skin

horny tissue (keratin), hard

sweat

death (cells, body)

fungus

thick

nail

COMBINING FORM

rhytid/o

EXAMPLE: **rhytid/ectomy**

COMBINING FORM

seb/o

EXAMPLE: **seb/o/rrhea**

COMBINING FORM

staphyl/o

EXAMPLE: **staphyl/o/coccus**

COMBINING FORM

strept/o

EXAMPLE: **strept/o/coccus**

COMBINING FORM

xer/o

EXAMPLE: **xer/o/derm/a**

PREFIX

epi-

EXAMPLE: **epi/derm/al**

PREFIX

intra-

EXAMPLE: **intra/derm/al**

PREFIX

para-

EXAMPLE: **par/onych/ia**

sebum (oil)

wrinkles

twisted chains

grapelike clusters

on, upon, over

dry, dryness

beside, beyond, around, abnormal

within

per-

EXAMPLE: per/cutane/ous

sub-

EXAMPLE: sub/cutane/ous

trans-

EXAMPLE: trans/derm/al

-a

EXAMPLE: pachy/o/derm/a

-coccus (pl. -cocci)

EXAMPLE: strept/o/coccus

-ectomy

EXAMPLE: rhytid/ectomy

-ia

EXAMPLE: par/onych/ia

-itis

EXAMPLE: dermat/itis

under, below

through

noun suffix, no meaning

through, across, beyond

excision or surgical removal

berry-shaped (form of bacterium)

inflammation

diseased or abnormal state, condition of

SUFFIX

-malacia

EXAMPLE: **onych/o/malacia**

SUFFIX

-opsy

EXAMPLE: **bi/opsy**

SUFFIX

-phagia

EXAMPLE: **onych/o/phagia**

SUFFIX

-plasty

EXAMPLE: **dermat/o/plasty**

SUFFIX

-rrhea

EXAMPLE: **seb/o/rrhea**

SUFFIX

-tome

EXAMPLE: **derma/tome**

COMBINING FORM

adenoid/o

EXAMPLE: **adenoid/itis**

COMBINING FORM

alveol/o

EXAMPLE: **alveol/itis**

view of, viewing

softening

surgical repair

eating or swallowing

instrument used to cut

flow, discharge

alveolus

adenoids

COMBINING FORM

atel/o

EXAMPLE: **atel/ectasis**

COMBINING FORM

bronchi/o, bronch/o

EXAMPLE: **bronchi/ectasis**

COMBINING FORM

capn/o

EXAMPLE: **capn/o/meter**

COMBINING FORM

diaphragmat/o, phren/o

EXAMPLE: **diaphragmat/o/cele**

COMBINING FORM

epiglott/o

EXAMPLE: **epiglott/itis**

COMBINING FORM

hem/o, hemat/o

EXAMPLE: **hem/o/thorax**

COMBINING FORM

laryng/o

EXAMPLE: **laryng/itis**

COMBINING FORM

lob/o

EXAMPLE: **lob/ectomy**

bronchus

imperfect, incomplete

diaphragm

carbon dioxide

blood

epiglottis

lobe

larynx

COMBINING FORM

muc/o

EXAMPLE: **muc/oid**

COMBINING FORM

nas/o, rhin/o

EXAMPLE: **rhin/o/plasty**

COMBINING FORM

orth/o

EXAMPLE: **orth/o/pnea**

COMBINING FORM

ox/i

EXAMPLE: **ox/i/meter**

COMBINING FORM

pharyng/o

EXAMPLE: **pharyng/itis**

COMBINING FORM

phon/o

EXAMPLE: **dys/phon/ia**

COMBINING FORM

pleur/o

EXAMPLE: **pleur/itis**

COMBINING FORM

**pneum/o,
pneumat/o,
pneumon/o**

EXAMPLE: **pneumon/ia**

nose

mucus

oxygen

straight

sound, voice

pharynx

lung, air

pleura

COMBINING FORM

pulmon/o

EXAMPLE: pulmon/ary

COMBINING FORM

py/o

EXAMPLE: py/o/thorax

COMBINING FORM

radi/o

EXAMPLE: radi/o/logy

COMBINING FORM

sept/o

EXAMPLE: sept/o/tomy

COMBINING FORM

sinus/o

EXAMPLE: sinus/o/tomy

COMBINING FORM

somn/o

EXAMPLE: poly/somn/o/graphy

COMBINING FORM

son/o

EXAMPLE: son/o/graphy

COMBINING FORM

spir/o

EXAMPLE: spir/o/meter

pus

lung

septum (wall off, fence)

x-rays, ionizing radiation

sleep

sinus

breathe, breathing

sound

COMBINING FORM

thorac/o

EXAMPLE: tonsill/itis

COMBINING FORM

tom/o

EXAMPLE: tom/o/graphy

COMBINING FORM

tonsill/o

EXAMPLE: tonsill/itis

COMBINING FORM

trache/o

EXAMPLE: trache/o/stomy

PREFIX

a-, an-

EXAMPLE: a/pnea

PREFIX

endo-

EXAMPLE: endo/scope

PREFIX

eu-

EXAMPLE: eu/pnea

PREFIX

poly-

EXAMPLE: poly/somn/o/graphy

to cut, section, or slice

thorax, chest, chest cavity

trachea

tonsil

within

absence of, without

many, much

normal, good

SUFFIX

-graph

EXAMPLE: radi/o/graph

SUFFIX

-graphy

EXAMPLE: poly/somn/o/graphy

SUFFIX

-meter

EXAMPLE: spir/o/meter

SUFFIX

-metry

EXAMPLE: spir/o/metry

SUFFIX

-pexy

EXAMPLE: pleur/o/pexy

SUFFIX

-pnea

EXAMPLE: a/pnea

SUFFIX

-rrhagia

EXAMPLE: rhin/o/rrhagia

SUFFIX

-scope

EXAMPLE: bronch/o/scope

process of recording,
radiographic imaging

instrument used to
record, the record

measurement

instrument used to
measure

breathing

surgical fixation,
suspension

instrument used for
visual examination

rapid flow of blood,
excessive bleeding

tachy-

EXAMPLE: tachy/pnea

-algia

EXAMPLE: thorac/algia

-ar, -ary, -eal

EXAMPLE: laryng/eal

-cele

EXAMPLE: pneumat/o/cele

-centesis

EXAMPLE: thorac/o/centesis

-ectasis

EXAMPLE: atel/ectasis

-emia

EXAMPLE: hyp/ox/emia

-gram

EXAMPLE: son/o/gram

pain

fast, rapid

hernia or protrusion

pertaining to

stretching out, dilation, expansion

surgical puncture to aspirate fluid (with a sterile needle)

the record, radiographic image

in the blood

-scopic

EXAMPLE: endo/scopic

-scopy

EXAMPLE: endo/scopy

-spasm

EXAMPLE: bronch/o/spasm

-stenosis

EXAMPLE: trache/o/stenosis

-stomy

EXAMPLE: laryng/o/stomy

-thorax

EXAMPLE: pneum/o/thorax

-tomy

EXAMPLE: trache/o/tomy

albumin/o

EXAMPLE: albumin/uria

visual examination

pertaining to visual examination

constriction or narrowing

sudden, involuntary muscle contraction

chest, chest cavity

creation of an artificial opening

albumin

cut into, incision

COMBINING FORM

azot/o

EXAMPLE: **azot/emia**

COMBINING FORM

blast/o

EXAMPLE: **nephr/o/blast/oma**

COMBINING FORM

cyst/o, vesic/o

EXAMPLE: **cyst/itis**

COMBINING FORM

glomerul/o

EXAMPLE: **glomerul/o/nephr/itis**

COMBINING FORM

glyc/o, glycos/o

EXAMPLE: **glycos/uria**

COMBINING FORM

hydr/o

EXAMPLE: **hydr/o/nephr/osis**

COMBINING FORM

lith/o

EXAMPLE: **lith/o/tripsy**

COMBINING FORM

meat/o

EXAMPLE: **meat/o/tomy**

developing cell,
germ cell

urea, nitrogen

glomerulus

bladder, sac

water

sugar

meatus (opening)

stone, calculus

COMBINING FORM

nephr/o, ren/o

EXAMPLE: ren/o/gram

COMBINING FORM

noct/i

EXAMPLE: noct/uria

COMBINING FORM

olig/o

EXAMPLE: olig/uria

COMBINING FORM

pyel/o

EXAMPLE: pyel/o/plasty

COMBINING FORM

ureter/o

EXAMPLE: ureter/o/stomy

COMBINING FORM

urethr/o

EXAMPLE: urethr/o/plasty

COMBINING FORM

urin/o, ur/o

EXAMPLE: urin/ary

SUFFIX

-iasis, -esis

EXAMPLE: nephr/o/lith/iasis

night

kidney

renal pelvis

scanty, few

urethra

ureter

condition

urine, urinary tract

SUFFIX

-lysis

EXAMPLE: **nephr/o/lysis**

SUFFIX

-ptosis

EXAMPLE: **nephr/o/ptosis**

SUFFIX

-rrhaphy

EXAMPLE: **cyst/o/rrhaphy**

SUFFIX

-tripsy

EXAMPLE: **lith/o/tripsy**

SUFFIX

-uria

EXAMPLE: **py/uria**

COMBINING FORM

andr/o

EXAMPLE: **andr/o/pathy**

COMBINING FORM

balan/o

EXAMPLE: **balan/itis**

COMBINING FORM

epididym/o

EXAMPLE: **epididym/ectomy**

drooping, sagging, prolapse

loosening, dissolution, separating

surgical crushing

suturing, repairing

male

urine, urination

epididymis

glans penis

orchid/o, orchi/o, orch/o

EXAMPLE: orchi/o/plasty

prostat/o

EXAMPLE: prostat/o/lith

sperm/o, spermat/o

EXAMPLE: olig/o/sperm/ia

vas/o

EXAMPLE: vas/ectomy

vesicul/o

EXAMPLE: vesicul/ectomy

-ism

EXAMPLE: an/orch/ism

arche/o

EXAMPLE: mcn/arche

cervic/o, trachel/o

EXAMPLE: cervic/itis

prostate gland

testis, testicle

vessel, duct (vas deferens in terms describing the male reproductive system)

sperm, spermatozoon

state of

seminal vesicle(s)

cervix

first, beginning

colp/o, vagin/o

EXAMPLE: **colp/o/perine/o/rrhaphy**

endometri/o

EXAMPLE: **endometri/osis**

episi/o, vulv/o

EXAMPLE: **episi/o/tomy**

gynec/o, gyn/o

EXAMPLE: **gynec/o/logist**

hymen/o

EXAMPLE: **hymen/o/tomy**

hyster/o, metr/o

EXAMPLE: **hyster/ectomy**

mamm/o, mast/o

EXAMPLE: **mast/ectomy**

men/o

EXAMPLE: **men/o/rrhagia**

endometrium

vagina

woman

vulva

uterus

hymen

menstruation

breast

oophor/o

EXAMPLE: oophor/ectomy

pelv/i

EXAMPLE: pelv/i/scopic

perine/o

EXAMPLE: perine/o/rrhaphy

salping/o

EXAMPLE: salping/o/cele

peri-

EXAMPLE: peri/metr/itis

-cleisis

EXAMPLE: colp/o/cleisis

-salpinx

EXAMPLE: hemat/o/salpinx

amni/o, amnion/o

EXAMPLE: amni/o/centesis

pelvis, pelvic bones,
pelvic cavity

ovary

uterine tube
(fallopian tube)

perineum

surgical closure

surrounding (outer)

amnion; amniotic fluid

uterine tube
(fallopian tube)

COMBINING FORM

cephal/o

EXAMPLE: micro/cephal/us

COMBINING FORM

chori/o

EXAMPLE: chori/o/carcin/oma

COMBINING FORM

embry/o

EXAMPLE: embry/o/genic

COMBINING FORM

esophag/o

EXAMPLE: esophag/eal

COMBINING FORM

fet/o, fet/i

EXAMPLE: fet/al

COMBINING FORM

gravid/o

EXAMPLE: nulli/gravid/a

COMBINING FORM

lact/o

EXAMPLE: lact/o/rrhea

COMBINING FORM

nat/o

EXAMPLE: neo/nat/o/logist

chorion

head

esophagus

embryo

pregnancy

fetus, unborn offspring

birth

milk

omphal/o

EXAMPLE: omphal/o/cele

par/o, part/o

EXAMPLE: par/a

prim/i

EXAMPLE: prim/i/gravid/a

pseud/o

EXAMPLE: pseud/o/cyesis

puerper/o

EXAMPLE: puerper/al

pylor/o

EXAMPLE: pylor/ic

terat/o

EXAMPLE: terat/o/gen

ante-, pre-

EXAMPLE: pre/nat/al

bear, give birth to, labor, childbirth

umbilicus, navel

false

first

pylorus, pyloric sphincter

childbirth

before

malformations

micro-

EXAMPLE: micro/cephal/us

multi-

EXAMPLE: multi/gravid/a

nulli-

EXAMPLE: nulli/par/a

post-

EXAMPLE: post/nat/al

-amnios

EXAMPLE: olig/o/hydr/amnios

-cyesis

EXAMPLE: pseud/o/cyesis

-e, -is, -us, -um

EXAMPLE: antc/part/um

-rrhexis

EXAMPLE: amni/o/rrhexis

many

small

after

pregnancy

amnion, amniotic fluid

rupture

noun suffix,
no meaning

-tocia

EXAMPLE: **dys/tocia**

angi/o

EXAMPLE: **angi/o/stenosis**

aort/o

EXAMPLE: **aort/o/gram**

arteri/o

EXAMPLE: **arteri/o/sclerosis**

ather/o

EXAMPLE: **ather/o/sclerosis**

atri/o

EXAMPLE: **atri/o/ventricul/ar**

cardi/o

EXAMPLE: **cardi/o/logist**

ech/o

EXAMPLE: **ech/o/cardi/o/gram**

vessel (usually refers to blood vessel)

birth, labor

artery

aorta

atrium

yellowish, fatty plaque

sound

heart

COMBINING FORM

electr/o

EXAMPLE: **electr/o/cardi/o/gram**

COMBINING FORM

isch/o

EXAMPLE: **isch/emia**

COMBINING FORM

lymph/o

EXAMPLE: **lymph/oma**

COMBINING FORM

lymphaden/o

EXAMPLE: **lymphaden/itis**

COMBINING FORM

myel/o

EXAMPLE: **myel/o/poiesis**

COMBINING FORM

phleb/o, ven/o

EXAMPLE: **intra/ven/ous**

COMBINING FORM

plasm/o

EXAMPLE: **plasm/apheresis**

COMBINING FORM

splen/o

EXAMPLE: **splen/o/megaly**

deficiency, blockage

electricity,
electrical activity

lymph node

lymph, lymph tissue

vein

bone marrow

spleen

plasma

COMBINING FORM

therm/o

EXAMPLE: hypo/therm/ia

COMBINING FORM

thromb/o

EXAMPLE: thromb/o/phleb/itis

COMBINING FORM

thym/o

EXAMPLE: thym/ectomy

COMBINING FORM

valv/o, valvul/o

EXAMPLE: valvul/o/plasty

COMBINING FORM

ventricul/o

EXAMPLE: atri/o/ventricul/ar

PREFIX

brady-

EXAMPLE: brady/card/ia

PREFIX

pan-

EXAMPLE: pan/cyt/o/penia

SUFFIX

-ac

EXAMPLE: cardi/ac

clot

heat

valve

thymus gland

slow

ventricle

pertaining to

all, total

-apheresis

EXAMPLE: plasm/apheresis

-penia

EXAMPLE: erythr/o/cyt/o/penia

-poiesis

EXAMPLE: myel/o/poiesis

-sclerosis

EXAMPLE: ather/o/sclerosis

abdomin/o, celi/o, lapar/o

EXAMPLE: abdomin/o/plasty

an/o

EXAMPLE: an/al

antr/o

EXAMPLE: antr/ectomy

append/o, appendic/o

EXAMPLE: appendic/itis

abnormal reduction
in number

removal

hardening

formation

anus

abdomen;
abdominal cavity

appendix

antrum

cec/o

EXAMPLE: ile/o/cec/al

cheil/o

EXAMPLE: cheil/o/plasty

chol/e

EXAMPLE: chol/e/cyst/o/gram

cholangi/o

EXAMPLE: cholangi/o/graphy

choledoch/o

EXAMPLE: choledoch/o/lith/iasis

col/o, colon/o

EXAMPLE: col/o/stomy

diverticul/o

EXAMPLE: diverticul/osis

duoden/o

EXAMPLE: duoden/al

lip(s)

cecum

bile duct(s)

gall, bile

colon

common bile duct

duodenum

diverticulum
(pl. diverticula) (pouch
extending from a
hollow organ)

COMBINING FORM

enter/o

EXAMPLE: gastr/o/enter/itis

COMBINING FORM

esophag/o

EXAMPLE: esophag/o/scope

COMBINING FORM

gastr/o

EXAMPLE: gastr/itis

COMBINING FORM

gingiv/o

EXAMPLE: gingiv/itis

COMBINING FORM

gloss/o, lingu/o

EXAMPLE: sub/lingu/al

COMBINING FORM

hepat/o

EXAMPLE: hepat/itis

COMBINING FORM

herni/o

EXAMPLE: herni/o/rrhaphy

COMBINING FORM

ile/o

EXAMPLE: ile/o/stomy

esophagus

intestine(s)
(small intestine)

gum(s)

stomach

liver

tongue

ileum

(protrusion of an organ
through a membrane
or cavity wall)

COMBINING FORM

jejun/o

EXAMPLE: gastr/o/jejun/o/stomy

COMBINING FORM

or/o, stomat/o

EXAMPLE: or/o/gastr/ic

COMBINING FORM

palat/o

EXAMPLE: palat/o/plasty

COMBINING FORM

pancreat/o

EXAMPLE: pancreat/itis

COMBINING FORM

peritone/o

EXAMPLE: peritone/al

COMBINING FORM

polyp/o

EXAMPLE: polyp/ectomy

COMBINING FORM

proct/o, rect/o

EXAMPLE: proct/o/logy

COMBINING FORM

pylor/o

EXAMPLE: pylor/o/plasty

mouth

jejunum

pancreas

palate

polyp, small growth

peritoneum

pylorus, pyloric
sphincter

rectum

sial/o

EXAMPLE: sial/o/lith

sigmoid/o

EXAMPLE: sigmoid/o/scopy

steat/o

EXAMPLE: steat/osis

uvul/o

EXAMPLE: uvul/ectomy

hemi-

EXAMPLE: hemi/col/ectomy

-pepsia

EXAMPLE: dys/pepsia

blephar/o

EXAMPLE: blephar/o/plasty

conjunctiv/o

EXAMPLE: conjunctiv/itis

sigmoid colon

saliva, salivary gland

uvula

fat

digestion

half

conjunctiva

eyelid

COMBINING FORM

cor/o, core/o, pupill/o

EXAMPLE: pupill/ary

COMBINING FORM

corne/o, kerat/o

EXAMPLE: corne/al

COMBINING FORM

cry/o

EXAMPLE: cry/o/retin/o/pexy

COMBINING FORM

cyst/o

EXAMPLE: dacry/o/cyst/itis

COMBINING FORM

dacry/o, lacrim/o

EXAMPLE: lacrim/al

COMBINING FORM

dipl/o

EXAMPLE: dipl/opia

COMBINING FORM

ir/o, irid/o

EXAMPLE: irid/o/plegia

COMBINING FORM

is/o

EXAMPLE: is/o/cor/ia

cornea

pupil

bladder, sac

cold

two, double

tear(s)

equal

iris

COMBINING FORM

ocul/o, ophthalm/o

EXAMPLE: **ophthalm/o/logy**

COMBINING FORM

opt/o

EXAMPLE: **opt/ic**

COMBINING FORM

phac/o, phak/o

EXAMPLE: **a/phak/ia**

COMBINING FORM

phot/o

EXAMPLE: **phot/o/phobia**

COMBINING FORM

retin/o

EXAMPLE: **retin/al**

COMBINING FORM

scler/o

EXAMPLE: **scler/o/malacia**

COMBINING FORM

ton/o

EXAMPLE: **ton/o/meter**

PREFIX

bi-, bin-

EXAMPLE: **bin/ocul/ar**

vision

eye

light

lens

sclera

retina

two

tension, pressure

-opia

EXAMPLE: **dipl/opia**

-phobia

EXAMPLE: **phot/o/phobia**

-plegia

EXAMPLE: **ophthalm/o/plegia**

audi/o

EXAMPLE: **audi/o/gram**

aur/i, ot/o

EXAMPLE: **ot/o/logy**

cochle/o

EXAMPLE: **cochle/ar**

labyrinth/o

EXAMPLE: **labyrinth/itis**

mastoid/o

EXAMPLE: **mastoid/itis**

abnormal fear of or aversion to specific things

vision (condition)

hearing

paralysis

cochlea

ear

mastoid bone

labyrinth

COMBINING FORM

myring/o

EXAMPLE: myring/o/plasty

COMBINING FORM

staped/o

EXAMPLE: staped/ectomy

COMBINING FORM

tympan/o

EXAMPLE: tympan/o/plasty

COMBINING FORM

vestibul/o

EXAMPLE: vestibul/ar

COMBINING FORM

ankyl/o

EXAMPLE: ankyl/osis

COMBINING FORM

aponeur/o

EXAMPLE: aponeur/o/rrhaphy

COMBINING FORM

arthr/o

EXAMPLE: arthr/itis

COMBINING FORM

burs/o

EXAMPLE: burs/itis

stapes

tympanic membrane
(eardrum)

vestibule

middle ear

aponeurosis

stiff, bent

bursa (cavity)

joint

COMBINING FORM

carp/o

EXAMPLE: carp/al

COMBINING FORM

chondr/o

EXAMPLE: chondr/ectomy

COMBINING FORM

clavic/o, clavicul/o

EXAMPLE: clavicul/ar

COMBINING FORM

cost/o

EXAMPLE: inter/cost/al

COMBINING FORM

crani/o

EXAMPLE: crani/al

COMBINING FORM

disk/o

EXAMPLE: disk/itis

COMBINING FORM

femor/o

EXAMPLE: femor/al

COMBINING FORM

fibul/o

EXAMPLE: fibul/ar

cartilage

carpals (wrist)

rib

clavicle (collarbone)

intervertebral disk

cranium (skull)

fibula (lower leg bone)

femur (upper leg bone)

humer/o

EXAMPLE: humer/al

ili/o

EXAMPLE: ili/o/femor/al

ischi/o

EXAMPLE: ischi/o/fibul/ar

kinesi/o

EXAMPLE: brady/kinesi/a

kyph/o

EXAMPLE: kyph/osis

lamin/o

EXAMPLE: lamin/ectomy

lord/o

EXAMPLE: lord/osis

lumb/o

EXAMPLE: lumb/o/sacr/al

ilium

humerus
(upper arm bone)

movement, motion

ischium

lamina (thin, flat plate
or layer)

hump

loin; lumbar region of
the spine

bent forward (increased
concavity of the spine)

mandibul/o

EXAMPLE: sub/mandibul/ar

maxill/o

EXAMPLE: maxill/itis

menisc/o

EXAMPLE: menisc/itis

my/o, myos/o

EXAMPLE: my/o/rrhaphy

myel/o

EXAMPLE: myel/oma

oste/o

EXAMPLE: oste/itis

patell/o

EXAMPLE: patell/ectomy

pelv/i

EXAMPLE: pelv/ic

maxilla (upper jawbone)

mandible
(lower jawbone)

muscle

meniscus (crescent)

bone

bone marrow

pelvis, pelvic bones,
pelvic cavity

patella (kneecap)

COMBINING FORM

petr/o

EXAMPLE: oste/o/petr/osis

COMBINING FORM

phalang/o

EXAMPLE: phalang/ectomy

COMBINING FORM

pub/o

EXAMPLE: pub/ic

COMBINING FORM

rachi/o, spondyl/o, vertebr/o

EXAMPLE: rachi/o/tomy

COMBINING FORM

radi/o

EXAMPLE: radi/al

COMBINING FORM

sacr/o

EXAMPLE: sacr/al

COMBINING FORM

sarc/o

EXAMPLE: oste/o/sarc/oma

COMBINING FORM

scapul/o

EXAMPLE: supra/scapul/ar

phalanx (pl. phalanges)
(any bone of the fingers
or toes)

stone

vertebra, spine,
vertebral column

pubis

sacrum

radius
(lower arm bone)

scapula (shoulder blade)

flesh, connective tissue

scoli/o

EXAMPLE: scoli/osis

stern/o

EXAMPLE: stern/o/clavicul/ar

synovi/o

EXAMPLE: synovi/ectomy

tars/o

EXAMPLE: tars/ectomy

ten/o, tend/o, tendin/o

EXAMPLE: tendin/itis

tibi/o

EXAMPLE: tibi/al

uln/o

EXAMPLE: uln/o/radi/al

inter-

EXAMPLE: inter/vertebr/al

sternum (breastbone)

(lateral) curved (spine)

tarsals (ankle bones)

synovia, synovial membrane

tibia (lower leg bone)

tendon

between

ulna (lower arm bone)

supra-

EXAMPLE: **supra/scapul/ar**

sym-, syn-

EXAMPLE: **sym/physis**

-asthenia

EXAMPLE: **my/asthenia**

-desis

EXAMPLE: **arthr/o/desis**

-physis

EXAMPLE: **sym/physis**

-schisis

EXAMPLE: **crani/o/schisis**

-trophy

EXAMPLE: **dys/trophy**

cerebell/o

EXAMPLE: **cerebell/itis**

together, joined

above

surgical fixation, fusion

weakness

split, fissure

growth

cerebellum

nourishment, development

cerebr/o

EXAMPLE: cerebr/al

dur/o

EXAMPLE: sub/dur/al

encephal/o

EXAMPLE: encephal/itis

esthesi/o

EXAMPLE: an/esthesi/a

gangli/o, ganglion/o

EXAMPLE: ganglion/ectomy

gli/o

EXAMPLE: gli/oma

mening/o, meningi/o

EXAMPLE: mening/o/cele

ment/o, psych/o

EXAMPLE: ment/al

hard, dura mater

cerebrum, brain

sensation, sensitivity, feeling

brain

glia

ganglion

mind

meninges

COMBINING FORM

mon/o

EXAMPLE: **mon/o/plegia**

COMBINING FORM

myel/o

EXAMPLE: **myel/o/graphy**

COMBINING FORM

neur/o

EXAMPLE: **neur/o/logist**

COMBINING FORM

phas/o

EXAMPLE: **dys/phas/ia**

COMBINING FORM

poli/o

EXAMPLE: **poli/o/myel/itis**

COMBINING FORM

quadr/i

EXAMPLE: **quadr/i/plegia**

COMBINING FORM

radic/o, radicul/o, rhiz/o

EXAMPLE: **radic/o/tomy**

SUFFIX

-iatrist

EXAMPLE: **psych/iatrist**

spinal cord (also means bone marrow)

one, single

speech

nerve

four

gray matter

specialist, physician

nerve root

-iatry

EXAMPLE: psych/iatry

-ictal

EXAMPLE: post/ictal

-paresis

EXAMPLE: hemi/paresis

acr/o

EXAMPLE: acr/o/megaly

adren/o, adrenal/o

EXAMPLE: adren/ectomy

calc/i

EXAMPLE: hyper/calc/emia

cortic/o

EXAMPLE: cortic/al

dips/o

EXAMPLE: poly/dips/ia

seizure, attack

treatment, specialty

extremities, height

slight paralysis

calcium

adrenal glands

thirst

cortex

endocrin/o

EXAMPLE: **endocrin/o/logist**

kal/i

EXAMPLE: **hypo/kal/emia**

natr/o

EXAMPLE: **hypo/natr/emia**

parathyroid/o

EXAMPLE: **parathyroid/oma**

pituitar/o

EXAMPLE: **hypo/pituitar/ism**

thyroid/o, thyr/o

EXAMPLE: **thyroid/ectomy**

-drome

EXAMPLE: **syn/drome**

potassium

endocrine

parathyroid glands

sodium

thyroid gland

pituitary gland

run, running

Recommended
Shelving Classification
Medical Terminology

9780323396479
CARDS: 978-0-323-39647-9

9780323396455
SET# 978-0-323-39645-5

ELSEVIER   elsevier.com